TABLE OF CONTENTS

INTRODUCTION

"Oh, I'm so glad I made it. I had no idea I could succeed "

Have you ever expressed a similar opinion?These and other remarks are made by people who have survived various deadly catastrophes.You can be grateful but also very anxious since there are important questions that need to be addressed. What about my close friends and family members? Are they safe? What possibilities does the feature offer me? Imagine this real-life scenario that has affected you, a recent incident that astonished and had an impact on the entire world, to help you better appreciate the gravity of this question. You undoubtedly avoided the plague. Covid-19, to be more specific. But keep in mind that everyone alive has a 100% probability of dying today because people still die at some time. This should serve as a reminder to us that we need to be more attentive about how we live.

Even though you managed to survive, you undoubtedly gained a lot of knowledge from that experience. But have you already forgotten everything that happened?

Remember that millions of people died as a result of this so soon. It's possible that you knew someone who passed away. There may even be family members present! Do you have a hard time forgetting the suffering you endured throughout this period?

Some people may have ignored safety procedures or just failed to pay attention. Keep in mind that ignoring a straightforward warning could be disastrous!

Never forget how important your life is! How quickly you decide to handle this circumstance could determine how tomorrow turns out for you!

CHAPTER ONE: LESSONS YOU DON'T FORGET SOON!

What have you discovered as a result of your escape? Escape from what? The recent COVID-19 that recently affected and almost ravaged the whole world. Don't forget that this resulted in millions of death. You may be acquainted with someone who passed away. Even your family members might be there! Do you find it easy to forget the pains that were experienced throughout this time? Paying attention to anything you might have neglected is crucial to your survival. Remember that disobeying a simple warning could be fatal!

Keep in mind that your life matters! Your tomorrow may depend on how urgently you choose to tackle this situation!

Many people perished. You witnessed it. In fact you keep wondering what might happen next. But eventually, life's realities start to sink in. You soon started feeling conflicted. You just so happened to pick yourself up among these survivors. Furthermore, you might recall experiencing the loss of loved ones. Or perhaps you stopped seeing those well-known faces because you learned that they perished in the pandemic. Such a loss. You start to worry how you would actually handle missing so many folks.

Is this all there is to life? You start to wonder how you even made it through among so many other issues. In fact, you were by far one of the most obedient people on Earth throughout these crucial pandemic moments. You followed all the COVID-19 regulations. But have you forgotten so quickly now that daily life has returned to normal?

Considering how you conduct your life each day will help you assess whether you have learned anything from the pandemic at this point in time. How frequently do you, for instance, wash your hands with soap and running water? Although a menial task, but it can prevent you from a fatal experience!

People consider washing their hands to be a pointless chore, but meditating on the seriousness of this simple task is your choice. There are many **reasons** people do not follow safety precautions. Some of those reasons are as follows:

Overconfidence

Overconfidence refers to a state of being overly confident or having an exaggerated sense of one's abilities, knowledge, or judgment. In the context of safety, overconfidence can lead individuals to believe that they are invulnerable to harm or that they can handle potentially dangerous situations without taking appropriate safety precautions. This can lead to a false sense of security and increase the risk of accidents or injuries. Overconfidence can also lead individuals to underestimate the potential consequences of not following safety protocols, which can put themselves and others at risk. It's important to recognize the potential dangers and take appropriate safety precautions to minimize the risks.

Lessons learned from overconfidence

Overconfidence can lead to negative outcomes, and there are several lessons we can learn from this:

Awareness: It is essential to be aware of our level of confidence and ensure that we are not underestimating the risks or overestimating our abilities. Being aware of our limitations can help us make better decisions.

Precaution: We should always take appropriate precautions, even when we feel confident in our abilities. Taking extra measures to ensure safety can help prevent accidents and injuries.

Humility: Recognizing that we don't know everything and being open to learning from others can help us avoid overconfidence. We should be willing to ask for help when we need it and seek out the advice of experts in areas where we may be less knowledgeable.

Risk assessment: We should conduct a thorough risk assessment before taking any action, particularly in situations where there may be potential danger. Understanding the risks and potential consequences can help us make more informed decisions.

Consequences: Finally, it is essential to recognize the potential consequences of our actions and take responsibility for any negative outcomes. Learning from our mistakes and taking steps to prevent them from happening again can help us avoid overconfidence in the future.

Misinformation:

People may have received inaccurate or misleading information about the risks or effectiveness of certain safety precautions.

Effects of misinformation on safety precautions

Misinformation can have significant negative effects on safety precautions. Here are some possible effects:

Decreased Compliance: Misinformation can lead to confusion and uncertainty about safety precautions. This can decrease compliance, as individuals may not understand which safety precautions to follow, or they may not believe that they are necessary.

Increased Risks: Misinformation can lead to individuals taking inappropriate safety measures or not taking safety precautions at all. This can increase the risks of accidents, injuries, and other safety hazards.

False Sense of Security: Misinformation can give individuals a false sense of security, leading them to believe that they are safe even when they are not. This can lead to complacency and an increased risk of accidents or injuries.

Lack of Trust: Misinformation can erode trust in safety precautions, safety regulations, and safety experts. This can make it harder to communicate important safety information and encourage individuals to follow safety precautions.

Delayed Response: Misinformation can lead to a delay in response to safety hazards or emergencies. This can increase the severity of accidents or injuries and make it

harder to mitigate the effects.

It is essential to address misinformation by providing

accurate information, educating individuals on safety

precautions, and encouraging compliance. Clear

communication, training, and consistent enforcement

can help mitigate the negative effects of misinformation

on safety precautions.

PROCRASTINATION

Procrastination is the act of delaying or postponing tasks or activities that should be done in a timely manner. Some, who lost their lives during the COVID-19, may have been privileged to live. If they had taken that urgent step to implement some information that were at their disposal, it could have saved their lives.

Is a common problem that can lead to decreased productivity and feelings of guilt, stress, and anxiety. To overcome procrastination, it can help to set clear goals, prioritize tasks, eliminate distractions, break down large tasks into smaller steps, and hold oneself accountable. Additionally, developing good time management habits, practicing self-discipline, and seeking support from others can also be helpful. Note that it will be good for you to understand clearly the effect of procrastination.

Effects of procrastination

Procrastination can have a variety of negative effects on an individual's life, including:

Decreased productivity: Delaying tasks leads to a backlog of work, which can make it difficult to complete everything on time.

Increased stress and anxiety: The longer a task is delayed, the more pressure there is to complete it, leading to feelings of stress and anxiety.

Decreased quality of work: Rushing to complete a task at the last minute often results in lower quality work.

Guilt and low self-esteem: Procrastination can lead to feelings of guilt and a negative self-image.

Missed opportunities: Delaying tasks can result in missed opportunities and deadlines.

Strained relationships: Procrastination can lead to missed deadlines and unfulfilled commitments, which can strain personal and professional relationships.

Overall, procrastination can have a negative impact on one's life, both personally and professionally. Taking steps to overcome procrastination and develop good time management habits can help to mitigate these effects. Having seen that all the effects are of no benefit, why not learn how to avoid it. It pays you better.

How to avoid procrastination

Here are some practical tips to avoid procrastination:

Set clear goals: Start by setting clear and achievable goals, and prioritize tasks that support these goals.

Break down tasks into smaller steps: Large tasks can seem overwhelming, but breaking them down into smaller, more manageable steps can make them less daunting.

Use a to-do list: Write down all the tasks you need to complete, and prioritize them based on importance and deadline.

Eliminate distractions: Identify and remove distractions, such as social media, emails, or television, that might interfere with your focus.

Use time-management techniques: Use techniques such as the Pomodoro method to stay on track and maximize productivity.

Hold yourself accountable: Set deadlines and hold yourself accountable for meeting them.

Practice self-discipline: Discipline yourself to stay focused on the task at hand and avoid distractions.

Obtain assistance: Surround yourself with positive individuals who will inspire and motivate you.

Remember, avoiding procrastination takes effort and practice, but with time, it can become a habit that leads to greater productivity and success.

Consequences of ignoring reminders

Ignoring reminders can have several consequences, including:

Missed deadlines or appointments: Neglecting reminders can lead to missing important deadlines or appointments, causing potential harm to one's personal or professional life.

Increased stress and anxiety: Consistently missing reminders can lead to a feeling of overwhelming responsibility and increase stress levels.

Decreased productivity: Ignoring reminders can make it difficult to prioritize tasks, leading to decreased productivity and inefficiency.

Negative impact on reputation: Failing to follow through on reminders can have a negative impact on one's reputation, potentially damaging personal and professional relationships.

Financial consequences: Ignoring reminders related to financial matters, such as paying bills, can result in late fees and other financial consequences.

Inconvenience:

 Safety precautions can sometimes be inconvenient or time-consuming, which may discourage people from following them. safety precautions due to inconvenience can lead to increased risks of accidents or injuries. Here are some lessons we can learn from this:

Importance: It is essential to understand the importance of safety precautions and how they can help prevent accidents and injuries. We should prioritize safety, even if it means taking extra time or effort.

Education: Providing education and training on the importance of safety precautions can help individuals understand why they are necessary and how they can be integrated into their work or daily routine.

Simplify: Simplifying safety procedures and making them easier to follow can help reduce the inconvenience factor. It can be useful to provide equipment or tools that make it easier to follow safety procedures or to develop checklists to help ensure that all necessary steps are taken.

Consequences: It is important to emphasize the potential consequences of not following safety precautions. When individuals understand the risks and potential consequences, they may be more likely to prioritize safety.

Encouragement: Encouraging individuals to take safety precautions and recognizing their efforts can help motivate them to prioritize safety. Positive reinforcement can be a powerful tool in promoting safe behavior.

Compliance: Finally, consistently enforcing safety regulations and guidelines can help ensure that individuals follow safety precautions, even if they are inconvenient. This can help create a culture of safety where individuals prioritize safety even when it is not easy or convenient.

Having a habit of ignoring reminders

Because of the imperfect nature of humans, we all need reminders at some points in our lives; especially life-saving ones. It is one thing to receive a reminder, but it is another thing to take serious what you have heard.

Consequences of Ignoring Reminders:

Ignoring reminders can have several consequences, including:

Missed deadlines or appointments: Neglecting reminders can lead to missing important deadlines or appointments, causing potential harm to one's personal or professional life.

Increased stress and anxiety: Consistently missing reminders can lead to a feeling of overwhelming responsibility and increase stress levels.

Decreased productivity: Ignoring reminders can make it difficult to prioritize tasks, leading to decreased productivity and inefficiency.

Negative impact on reputation: Failing to follow through on reminders can have a negative impact on one's reputation, potentially damaging personal and professional relationships.

Financial consequences: Ignoring reminders related to financial matters, such as paying bills, can result in late fees and other financial consequences.

What ever, the reason(s), failure to follow life saving directives is always disastrous as many life experiences had shown. If it is possible to reverse the hand of clock, many people who took rash decisions and ignored warning signed would surely want to correct their wrongs. So ask yourself: " what have I learned from the recent Pandemic that I must not fail to implement to keep living?" That's a question for meditation.

Many people blamed the media for the perils they went through, especially during covid-19. Some even claimed that at a certain point, they even ignored the Media completely. How do you view the media?

CHAPTER TWO: FRESH LOOK AT NEWS MEDIA

Three friends�James, Jack, and Jerry�were sent by the company they work with to the Golden City to do some population research. They have a deadline for submitting their assignments. They were instructed, among other things, to give the news media precedence. Although less significant, this instruction is nonetheless important. James disregarded that information, since he had lost all faith in the media as a result of one inaccurate report about it. Jack found some important information in the media, but he didn't do anything with it. He just shrugged it off. As for Jerry, he found it difficult to consistently listen to the news, but he made an effort to do so and followed all the instructions he received in connection with his tasks in the Golden City from the news media. With what result? In the end, Jerry was the only one who completed that task successfully. Regarding the other two, they nearly lost their lives while working there just because they disobeyed instructions. The purpose of this scenario is to show how people perceive the media.

WHAT NEWS MEDIA IS ALL ABOUT

News media refers to the outlets and platforms (such as newspapers, television and radio stations, online news websites, etc.) that provide news and information to the public. The primary purpose of news media is to gather, report, and disseminate information about events and issues of public interest. This can include local, national, and international news, as well as stories on politics, sports, entertainment, science and technology, health, and other topics. News media also serves as a watchdog, holding those in power accountable for their actions and exposing wrongdoing, and promoting public debate and understanding of important issues. The ultimate goal of news media is to inform, educate, and engage the public, enabling citizens to make informed decisions and participate in the democratic process.

ROLES OF MEDIA IN HISTORY

Media has played a crucial role in shaping history. Throughout history, the media has been used as a powerful tool to inform, educate, entertain, and even manipulate the masses. Here are some of the key roles that media has played in history:

Spreading information: The media has been instrumental in disseminating news and information to the masses, especially in times of war and political upheaval. From newspapers to radio and television, the media has provided a means for people to stay informed about what is happening in the world.

Creating public opinion: Media has also been a powerful force in shaping public opinion. Through editorial content, opinion pieces, and investigative reporting, the media has the power to sway public sentiment on issues ranging from politics to social justice.

Propaganda: In times of war and political unrest, the media has often been used to spread propaganda and misinformation. Governments and other organizations have used the media to shape public opinion and to control the narrative.

Entertainment: The media has played a significant role in providing entertainment to people throughout history.

From books and plays to movies and television, the media has offered an escape from the stresses of daily life.

Education: Media has been a valuable source of education and learning throughout history. From books and newspapers to educational programs on television and online, the media has helped to disseminate knowledge and information to people around the world.

Holding power accountable: The media has been an important watchdog of power, calling attention to corruption and abuses of power by governments and other organizations. Investigative reporting and exposés have helped to uncover and shed light on issues that might otherwise have gone unnoticed.

Overall, the media has played a critical role in shaping history, from spreading information and creating public opinion to serving as a tool for propaganda and entertainment.

WHY SOME HAVE LOST INTEREST IN THE NEWS MEDIA

There are several reasons why some people have lost interest in news media:

Perception of bias: Many people believe that the news media has a political bias and is not presenting a balanced view of the issues. This can lead to a loss of trust in the news media.

Overload of information: With the rise of the internet and social media, people are exposed to an overwhelming amount of information and news. This can make it difficult for people to differentiate between credible and credible sources, leading to skepticism and disinterest.

Sensationalism: Some news media outlets have a tendency to focus on sensational stories and events, rather than important issues and facts. This can lead to a feeling of being inundated with "fake news" or sensationalized stories.

Decreased credibility: There have been instances of fake news and misinformation being spread through news media, which has contributed to a decrease in credibility and trust in the news media.

Alternative sources: With the rise of social media and other alternative sources of information, people are increasingly turning to these platforms for their news and information, which may be less credible but more personalized and appealing to individual interests.

All of these factors contribute to a declining interest in traditional news media and a shift towards more personalized sources of information. Despite all these reasons given, it would be nice to examine the benefits of news media.

Benefits of news media

News media has several benefits, including:

Information dissemination: News media provides a platform for the dissemination of information to a large audience in a timely and efficient manner.

Holding the powerful accountable: News media acts as a watchdog, holding those in power accountable for their actions, and exposing corruption and wrongdoings.

Promoting public debate: News media helps promote public debate on important issues, encouraging citizens to form informed opinions and participate in the democratic process.

Supporting local communities: Local news media outlets can provide important information about events and issues in a community, as well as promoting local businesses and cultural events.

Emergency alerts: News media can provide crucial information and updates during emergencies, helping to keep people informed and safe.

THE BEST WAY TO BENEFIT FROM THE NEWS MEDIA

To benefit from the news media, it's important to follow a few key principles:

Seek out multiple sources: In order to get a well-rounded understanding of an issue, it's important to gather information from multiple sources. This can help to reduce the influence of bias and provide a more complete picture of the situation.

Verify information: With the prevalence of misinformation and fake news, it's important to verify information from credible sources before accepting it as truth. This can involve fact-checking and checking multiple sources to confirm a story's accuracy.

Engage with diverse perspectives: Exposure to different perspectives and opinions can help to broaden your understanding of an issue and promote critical thinking.

Avoid sensationalism: Stay away from news sources that focus on sensational stories, and instead seek out sources that provide in-depth coverage of important issues.

Take a break: It's important to limit your exposure to the news and take breaks from consuming news content, especially if you feel overwhelmed or stressed by the information being presented.

In a summary, do not be gullible to all information you get from the media.Rather, verify every information you consider vital for your own consumption.

By following these principles, you can benefit from the news media by staying informed on important issues, engaging with diverse perspectives, and maintaining a healthy relationship with the information being presented. Remember how it turned out for James, Jack and Jerry!

It would be reasonable to comprehend the concept of the human body for a healthy lifestyle having observed the necessity to not forget the lesson gained from the recent pandemic and having a clearer picture of the media. Keep in mind that a healthy person would take the necessary steps to keep that appearance. If you don't feel well, you should be vigilant at all times!

CHAPTER THREE: UNDERSTANDING THE PRINCIPLE OF HUMAN BODY FOR A HEALTHY LIVING

Healthy living is another vital issue that people fail to take note off. Throughout the history of modern science, scientists have tried to understand the principles that govern the operation of the human body. Guess what? The results emerging from their research are have helped to save lots of life.

Despite its importance, some of the principles of the human body are often ignored or overlooked by individuals, leading to negative health consequences.

Some examples include:

Ignoring the importance of physical activity: Many people do not understand the importance of regular exercise for maintaining good health, and may engage in sedentary lifestyles that lead to weight gain, cardiovascular disease, and other health problems.

Overlooking the importance of nutrition: People may not realize the impact of their diet on their health and well-being, and may consume unhealthy or imbalanced diets that lead to deficiencies, chronic diseases, and other health problems.

Neglecting the importance of sleep: Sleep is essential for restoring and repairing the body, but many people do not understand its importance and may neglect their sleep in favor of other activities.

Failing to manage stress: People may not understand the impact of chronic stress on their health and may neglect to manage it effectively, leading to chronic stress-related conditions such as anxiety, depression, and cardiovascular disease.

Ignoring the importance of mental and emotional well-being: People may overlook the importance of mental and emotional well-being for overall health and may neglect to engage in activities that promote good mental health, such as mindfulness, meditation, and social connection.

By understanding and embracing the principles of the human body, individuals can make informed decisions about their health and wellness and improve their quality of life.

The human body is based on several key principles that include:

Anatomy and Physiology: The structure and function of the body's organs and systems, including the skeleton, muscles, cardiovascular, respiratory, digestive, nervous and endocrine systems.

Homeostasis: The ability of the body to maintain stability and balance in its internal environment, despite changes in the external environment.

Metabolism: The chemical processes that occur within the body to maintain life, including the conversion of food into energy and the elimination of waste products.

Cellular organization: The basic unit of life in the body is the cell, and cells are organized into tissues, organs, and systems that work together to carry out specific functions.

Adaptation and response: The body has the ability to respond and adapt to internal and external stimuli, including physical activity, stress, and disease.

Growth and Development: The body changes and grows over time, with different stages of development occurring in childhood, adolescence, and adulthood.

IMPORTANCE OF UNDERSTANDING PRINCIPLE OF HUMAN BODY

Understanding the principles of the human body is important for several reasons, including:

Health and Wellness: Understanding the basic principles of anatomy, physiology, and metabolism can help individuals make informed decisions about their health and wellness, including nutrition, exercise, and stress management.

Clinical Practice: Health professionals, such as doctors, nurses, and physiotherapists, need a deep understanding of the human body to diagnose and treat illnesses and injuries effectively.

Research and Development: A deeper understanding of the human body helps researchers to develop new medical treatments, technologies, and medications to improve health and prevent disease.

Personal growth: Understanding how the body works and what it needs to function optimally can help individuals make positive changes in their lifestyle and habits.

Appreciation of the human body: A deeper understanding of the human body can lead to greater appreciation for its complex and amazing abilities, and

for the importance of taking care of oneself.

Overall, understanding the principles of the human body

is crucial for promoting good health, advancing medical

knowledge and technology, and fostering personal

growth and well-being.

Eating a balanced diet: Many people have a tendency to

eat junk food or processed food, which is high in sugar,

salt, and unhealthy fats.

Exercising regularly: Lack of physical activity is a common

issue, especially among people who have sedentary jobs.

Getting enough sleep: Many people have busy lifestyles and sacrifice sleep for work or leisure activities.

Managing stress: Many people ignore the importance of managing stress and do not practice stress-reducing techniques.

Avoiding smoking and limiting alcohol consumption: Despite being aware of the harmful effects, many people continue to smoke and consume excessive amounts of alcohol.

Maintaining a healthy weight: People often ignore the importance of maintaining a healthy weight and may not be aware of their body mass index (BMI).

Staying hydrated: People often forget to drink enough water and may rely on sugary drinks instead.

Getting regular check-ups: Some people avoid going to the doctor and neglect their health.

Practicing safe habits: People may neglect safety precautions, such as wearing sunscreen or using seat belts, which can put their health at risk.

Eat a balanced and nutritious diet: Include a variety of fruits, vegetables, whole grains, and lean protein sources. Limit processed foods, sugar, and saturated fats.

Exercise regularly: Aim for at least 30 minutes of physical activity per day, such as walking, running, cycling, or swimming.

Get enough sleep: Aim for 7–9 hours of sleep per night to promote physical and mental well-being.

Manage stress: Practice stress-reducing techniques such as meditation, yoga, or deep breathing.

Avoid smoking and limit alcohol consumption: Both smoking and excessive alcohol consumption are harmful to your health.

Maintain a healthy weight: Keep track of your weight and body mass index (BMI) and work to maintain a healthy range.

Stay hydrated: Drink plenty of water throughout the day to stay hydrated and support your overall health.

Practice safe habits: Wear sunscreen, use seat belts, and follow other safety precautions to protect your health.

CHAPTER FOUR:UNDERSTANDING COMPREHENSIVE HEALTH

To live and enjoy life, we all desire to be in excellent health. The greatest influence on how long and how well we live may come from what we know about comprehensive health and how we choose to apply that knowledge. It is recommended to pay close attention to the essential components of overall health. One of the best things we could do is to take note of and implement these suggestions!

Comprehensive health is a term used to describe a comprehensive approach to wellbeing that considers social, environmental, and environmental aspects in addition to physical health. It is a thorough method of health and wellbeing that considers a person as a whole rather than concentrating on just one area of fitness.

PHYSICAL WELLBEING

Physical health is the status of a person's physique and their capacity to go about their daily lives without pain or restriction. It covers a range of topics, including overall fitness, strength, flexibility, and endurance. Healthy eating habits, regular exercise, and the absence of significant chronic ailments are characteristics of someone in good physical health. Regular doctor visits, getting adequate sleep, controlling stress, and abstaining from harmful habits like smoking and binge-drinking are

all part of maintaining excellent physical health.

HOW A NUTRITIOUS DIET HELPS MAINTAIN PHYSICAL HEALTH

By giving the body the nutrition and energy it needs to function correctly, a nutritious diet can help promote good physical health. Maintaining a healthy weight, preventing chronic illnesses including heart disease, diabetes, and some malignancies, and boosting the immune system are all benefits. A diet high in fruits, vegetables, whole grains, lean protein, and healthy fats can support the development and repair of tissues in the body as well as promote good skin, hair, and nails.

Limiting processed meals, added sugars, and saturated fats can also help lower the chance of developing chronic illnesses and enhance general physical health.

How exercise on a daily basis helps maintain healthy health

By enhancing cardiovascular fitness, preserving a healthy weight, and strengthening muscles and bones, regular exercise can improve overall health. Additionally, it can lower the risk of developing chronic conditions like heart disease, type 2 diabetes, and several types of cancer. Stress, anxiety, and sadness can all be reduced by exercise, which also benefits mental health. Exercise has also been found to enhance cognitive performance and postpone the onset of age-related cognitive decline. In general, frequent exercise is a crucial component of a healthy lifestyle and can enhance general wellbeing.

HOW A LACK OF CHRONIC DISEASE BENEFITS ONE'S HEALTH

A vital aspect of excellent health is the absence of chronic disease. Chronic conditions can significantly affect a person's quality of life and general well-being, including heart disease, diabetes, and several malignancies. They may also be expensive in terms of medical costs and lost wages. People can live active, full lives free from the restrictions and consequences that these illnesses can bring about by avoiding chronic illnesses. Furthermore, avoiding chronic conditions can reduce the risk of dying too soon.

Preventive actions including consistent exercise, a nutritious diet, and quitting smoking can minimize advantages of physical fitness

Having good physical health has various advantages, including:

Improved life quality and general well-being.

Increased vigor and endurance.

Improved sleep

decreased risk of developing chronic conditions like diabetes, heart disease, and some types of cancer.

Stronger immune system, which can aid in the resistance to diseases and infections.

Improved mental health and mood.

Improved coordination and balance, which can help stop falls and injuries.

Increased capacity to carry out daily tasks and keep one's independence as one becomes older.

Increased physical stress tolerance, such as while moving large goods or doing hard labor.

Better self-esteem and physical appearance.

A happy and satisfying existence generally depends on having good physical health.

EFFECTS OF DISREGARDING PHYSICAL HEALTH

Negative effects of neglecting physical health include a higher risk of developing chronic conditions like obesity, type 2 diabetes, heart disease, and some types of cancer. As well as reducing mobility and danger of injury, it can also make it harder to carry out daily tasks. Additionally, poor physical health can have a detrimental effect on general quality of life and mental health. Moreover, it may result in higher healthcare expenses.

MENTAL HEALTH

The ability of a person to process and deal with their emotions in a healthy and adaptive way is referred to as emotional health. It includes elements like:

Emotional stability is the capacity to maintain a constant, even emotional state, as well as the ability to properly control and regulate one's emotions. Being even-tempered, cool, and capable of handling stress and challenging situations in a constructive and positive way are characteristics of it. In general, emotionally secure people are better equipped to establish and sustain healthy relationships and feel better all around.

Self-awareness:

Self-awareness is the capacity of a person to be aware of and comprehend their own feelings, ideas, and mental states. It also entails the capacity to comprehend one's own existence and the effects of one's deeds on both oneself and others. Self-awareness is seen as a higher-order cognitive function in cognitive psychology that is connected to introspection and metacognition. Some researchers have also asserted that one of the core components of consciousness is self-awareness.

Personal pride:

Self-esteem is a person's total perception of their own value or self-worth. It is how someone views themselves, their skills, and their overall value as a person. While those with low self-esteem may feel bad about themselves and their skills, those with high self-esteem typically have a positive self-image and confidence in their talents. Experiences, interpersonal interactions, and outside criticism from others are all factors that might have an impact on one's sense of self. In therapy and personal development, raising one's self-esteem is frequently the objective.

Resilience is the capacity of an individual to deal with and bounce back from trying circumstances, such as stress, trauma, adversity, or change. It is the ability to overcome failures, adapt and advance in the face of difficulties. A multifaceted concept, resilience is influenced by psychological, social, and biological variables. It can be created and strengthened through time by using a variety of techniques, such as creating a solid support system, learning how to cope, reflecting on the past, maintaining a positive outlook, exercising regularly, and maintaining good bodily and mental health. Considered to be a key safeguard for both physical and mental health, resilience.

The capacity to comprehend and control one's own emotions as well as those of others is a sign of excellent emotional health. They have the capacity to make and keep wholesome relationships, create and achieve goals, and adjust to change.

A person who is in good emotional health is able to manage life's everyday challenges, work efficiently, and make significant contributions to their community. Additionally, it conveys the ability to overcome obstacles and bounce back from trying circumstances.

In order to maintain excellent mental health, one must also look after their physical needs, get enough sleep, practice self-care, and ask for assistance when required. In the event that professional assistance is required, it also entails visiting a therapist, counselor, or psychologist if you're in emotional distress.

ADVANTAGES OF MENTAL HEALTH

There are many advantages to having excellent mental health, and these advantages can be beneficial in all facets of life. Among the advantages are:

Increased capacity to handle stress and hardship.

Improved connections with friends, family, and coworkers.

Increased sentiments of joy, contentment, and satisfaction with life in general.

A greater sense of self-awareness and self-worth.

Improved capacity for decision-making and problem-solving.

Improved capacity for setting and achieving goals.

Enhanced assertiveness and communication abilities.

Increased capacity for appropriate emotion control and expression.

Greater capacity for resiliency and recovery from adversity.

Enhanced physical health, since there is a link between mental and physical wellness.

Overall, a happy and meaningful life depends on having good emotional health. It can assist people in establishing and maintaining healthy relationships, achieving their ambitions, and discovering meaning and purpose in their life.

SOCIAL HEALTH

The ability to engage with others in a healthy and constructive way is referred to as social health. It includes skills like empathy, communication, and the capacity to establish and keep good relationships. A person who has good social health is able to establish and keep wholesome bonds with their loved ones, friends, and others of their community. They are able to sympathize with people and express their views and feelings clearly.

It's important to practice empathy and understanding as well as effective emotion expression if you want to maintain healthy social health. It also entails creating a solid network of family and friends, as well as getting active in pursuits and groups that share one's beliefs and passions. Creating and sustaining solid social networks can offer psychological support, useful help, and a sense of community.

A strong social network is crucial for general wellbeing because it can provide people a sense of purpose, raise their self-esteem, and open doors for personal development. Strong social ties have been linked to longer lifespans and improved physical and mental health, according to studies.

Social health is important.

For a number of reasons, social health is crucial to overall wellbeing.

Strong social ties can give people a sense of belonging, practical support, and emotional support.

They may provide people a feeling of direction and significance in their lives.

They can raise one's sense of worth and self-esteem.

Furthermore, they may present chances for one's personal development.

Social relationships are associated in a lower risk of depression, anxiety, and other mental health conditions, therefore they can enhance mental health.

They can enhance physical health because strong social ties are associated with stronger immune systems, lower blood pressure, and a lower risk of developing chronic illnesses like heart disease and stroke.

Social ties are associated with a stronger capacity to deal with stress and adversity, therefore they can increase resilience.

They can foster a sense of belonging to the community as well as safety and security.

In general, social relationships are crucial to our lives and wellbeing. They give us a sense of community and purpose while assisting us in overcoming life's obstacles. Positive outlooks on life and improved stress and adversity coping skills are characteristics of people with good social health.

SPIRITUAL HEALTH

Spiritual health refers to an individual's sense of purpose, connection to something greater than oneself, and the ability to find meaning and fulfillment in life. It encompasses aspects such as values, beliefs, and faith. A person with good spiritual health has a sense of meaning and purpose in their life, and is able to find hope and peace in difficult situations. They may have a sense of connection to something greater than themselves, whether that be a higher power, nature, or a sense of interconnectedness with others.

Praying, journaling, or spending time in nature are all examples of spiritual health-promoting activities. It may also entail establishing ties with a group of like-minded people, such as a religious or spiritual organization. It's a unique journey that is both personal and subjective and might vary from person to person. Religion can be a source of spiritual health for some people, but it can also be found in nature, the arts, or close relationships.

A sense of meaning and purpose, as well as a sense of optimism and calm, may all be derived from having a healthy spiritual life, which is crucial for general wellbeing. It can aid people in finding meaning and hope in trying circumstances, and assist them in making sense of their surroundings. According to studies, those who hold strong spiritual convictions typically have better mental health and are better equipped to handle stress and adversity.

THE HEALTH BENEFITS OF SPIRITUAL HEALTH

A sense of meaning, purpose, and connection to something more than oneself can be fostered by having a healthy spiritual life. Additionally, it may result in a stronger sense of inner tranquility and a more upbeat attitude on life. Besides, spiritual practices like meditation and prayer can enhance general wellbeing and assist both physical and mental health by lowering stress, anxiety, and despair.

INTELLECTUAL FITNESS

The term "intellectual health" refers to a person's capacity for critical and creative thought, as well as their capacity for lifelong learning and growth. It includes skills like problem-solving, judgment, and the capacity to learn and use knowledge. A person with strong intellectual functioning is able to learn and use new information, think critically and creatively, and think creatively. They have an open-minded, inquisitive mind that is constantly learning and developing.

Being curious and inquisitive, questioning one's views, and taking part in activities that foster learning and progress are all part of maintaining healthy intellectual health. This can involve engaging in things like reading, picking up a new interest or talent, having intriguing conversations, or seeing new places. It also entails questioning one's own beliefs and seeking out other viewpoints.

A sense of personal growth and self-awareness, as well as the capacity to make wise decisions and solve difficulties, may all be attributed to having good intellectual health, which is crucial for overall wellbeing. It can aid people in navigating and making sense of the complex environment they find themselves in.

According to studies, those who participate in intellectually stimulating activities typically have better mental health and are better equipped to handle stress and adversity.

GROWTH OF INTELLECTUAL HEALTH

Reading: Increasing your knowledge and comprehension of a variety of subjects can be accomplished by reading books, articles, and other publications.

Learning: To gain new knowledge or skills in a particular profession, enroll in seminars, workshops, or online courses.

Writing: Expressing your thoughts and ideas clearly through writing in a journal, blog, or other written content will help you communicate more effectively.

To improve your critical thinking abilities, practice studying and evaluating facts, claims, and viewpoints.

Work on solving riddles, puzzles, and other brainteasers to hone your problem-solving skills.

Creativity: To increase your creativity and imagination, try acting, writing, music, or other creative pursuits.

Socializing: Engage in conversation, join a club or group, and interact with others to develop your social and interpersonal abilities.

To guarantee you have ample time for mental and intellectual interests, prioritize your tasks and manage your time well.

Reflect on your thoughts, feelings, and deeds on a regular basis to better understand yourself.

Exercise, a balanced diet, and enough sleep are all essential for preserving physical health, which is necessary for maintaining mental and intellectual well-being.

the significance of mental health

For various reasons, intellectual health is crucial to overall wellbeing.

It may result in a feeling of self-awareness and personal development.

It enables people to solve issues successfully and make educated decisions.

It can aid people in navigating and making sense of the complex environment around them.

It can enhance cognitive performance and guard against cognitive aging.

It may improve feelings of worth and self-esteem.

It can increase focus and memory.

It may encourage originality and thoughtfulness.

It might provide people a sense of fulfillment and purpose.

Intellectual stimulation is associated with a lower incidence of depression and cognitive decline, therefore it can help with mental health.

It can raise life quality in general.

In general, mental health is a crucial component of general wellbeing. It enables people to keep learning throughout their lives, to develop, and to comprehend the world around them. In addition to fostering a sense of personal progress and self-awareness, it can assist people in navigating the complexity of the world around them and helping them make wise judgments.

You should be concerned about the future now that you have the knowledge you need to live a healthy lifestyle and know other essential facts for survival.

CHAPTER FIVE: GET READY FOR THE UNTHINKABLE

Despite the fact that the pandemic was passed. Natural disasters continue to present mankind with some major problems. These catastrophes have undoubtedly always happened throughout the history of humanity, but this time they are more severe.

Natural catastrophes include phenomena like earthquakes, hurricanes, and tornadoes that are brought on by natural forces. These occurrences have the potential to significantly affect people, communities, and the environment, as well as result in property damage and fatalities. It would be acceptable to inquire whether the Pandemic qualifies as a natural disaster before going over some common natural disasters.

Is the pandemic a natural disaster?

A pandemic is not considered a natural disaster in the traditional sense. Natural disasters, such as hurricanes, earthquakes, and tsunamis, are events caused by natural forces that can result in widespread destruction, loss of life, and other impacts. Pandemics, on the other hand, are caused by the spread of infectious diseases, which are primarily driven by human activity and behavior, rather than natural forces. However, both natural disasters and pandemics can have significant impacts on societies, including loss of life, economic disruption, and changes to the way people live and work. Therefore, some experts have described pandemics as a type of "human-caused disaster." Regardless of the specific classification, pandemics and natural disasters both highlight the importance of preparedness and response planning, as well as the need for continued research and investment in public health and safety.

The following are examples of typical natural disasters:

(a) Earthquakes: The shifting of tectonic plates in the earth's crust is what causes earthquakes. They have the potential to create landslides, tsunamis, and damage to infrastructure and structures.

(b) Hurricanes: Hurricanes are tropical storms that develop over the Atlantic Ocean and have the potential to cause flooding, strong winds, and heavy rain in coastal regions.

(c) Tornadoes: Tornadoes are ferocious windstorms that can seriously harm infrastructure and structures. Although they can happen anywhere in the world, they frequently happen in the Midwest of the United States.

(d) Wildfires: Large fires with the potential to spread quickly and devastate homes, structures, and natural habitats are known as "wildfires." They are frequently brought on by arid weather, powerful gusts, and lightning.

(e) Floods: Floods can seriously harm homes, structures, and infrastructure. They are brought on by heavy rain or by dam or levee failure.

It is important for people to be prepared for natural disasters by having an emergency plan in place and keeping supplies such as food, water, and first aid kits on hand. It is also important for communities to have emergency response systems in place to help mitigate the impact of natural disasters

You can take the following actions to get ready for natural disasters:

1. Understand the risks: Conduct research on the different categories of natural disasters that are most prevalent in your area.

2. Create a plan: Create an emergency plan with a list of essential supplies and documents, evacuation routes, and a communication strategy.

3. Put together a kit: Always have a supply of non-perishable food, water, first aid supplies, and other necessities on hand.

4. Stay informed: Keep up with local news, weather reports, and emergency alerts to stay informed about the weather and other potential natural disasters.

5. Ensure the safety of your property: Take precautions to ensure the safety of your property by securing loose items outside, installing shutters or storm windows, and strengthening your roof and foundation.

6. Be prepared: Become knowledgeable about emergency procedures, including how to shut off utilities and where to find shelter.

7. Get involved: Take part in emergency preparedness training or think about joining a neighborhood association.

In the event of a natural disaster, by taking these precautions, you may help protect your safety and the safety of your family.

CHAPTER SIX: DO NOT QUICKLY FORGET YESTERDAY

Time sure flies. This is what the majority of individuals remark while recalling experiences when viewing a photograph, reading a letter, or taking part in activities related to those events. It could be a period of introspection or something else. But the most important query is, "What have I learned from this memory?" If, honestly, it hasn't imparted any lessons—whether positive or negative—then don't bother trying to remember them. Of course, there are a number of circumstances that may make it easier to forget the past, such as:

Interference: This occurs when new information interferes with the retrieval of old memories, causing them to fade.

Decay: Over time, memories may fade and become less accessible due to the physical changes in the brain that occur during memory formation and storage.

Retroactive Interference: This occurs when newly learned information causes older memories to become less accessible.

Proactive Interference: This occurs when previously learned information interferes with the recall of new information.

Emotional state: Emotional experiences and stress can have a significant impact on memory, causing some events to be remembered more vividly while others are forgotten.

Sleep deprivation: Lack of sleep can have a negative effect on memory, making it harder to recall past events.

Alcohol or drug use: Substance abuse can impair memory and make it difficult to recall past events.

Brain damage or injury: Physical damage to the brain, such as from a head injury, can affect memory and make it harder to recall past events. What ever the case, we should not fail to learn from the past for the sake of our feature.

Whatever the situation, the facts still remain that we must always be prepared for any emergency we encounter. While being careful, we need not play with information gotten from the right source in the news

Media.

CONCLUSION

We have no choice but to adapt to the greatest way of life because we live in a world where unforeseen occurrences are going to happen! We should never stop remembering that unexpected things happen in our world, even when we manage to avert any calamity. With that in mind, we can always draw lessons from the past and plan ahead, especially by taking all the necessary steps to lead a healthy life and following safety directives promptly. Our commitment to the correct news sources is crucial to our ability to be informed about events in the world around us and maintain our safety. The right outcome is produced by doing the right thing at the appropriate moment.